Lose Weight, Feel Great

THE JOURNEY BEGINS

Losing weight can be a challenging but rewarding journey. It requires dedication, commitment, and a healthy approach to lifestyle changes. This book will guide you through the process, providing you with the knowledge and tools you need to achieve your weight loss goals.

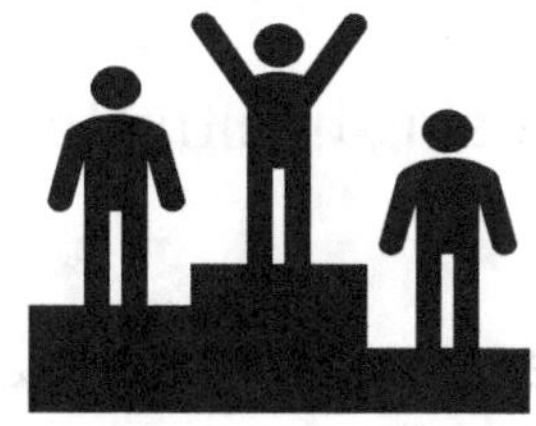

By/ Fouad Elqutamy

Chapter 1: Understanding Weight Loss

- The science of weight loss: metabolism, calories, and hormones

- Setting realistic goals: short-term and long-term targets

- Overcoming common misconceptions: fad diets and quick fixes

Chapter 2: Making Lifestyle Changes

- Nutrition basics: macronutrients, micronutrients, and portion control

- Meal planning and preparation: healthy recipes and time-saving tips

- Hydration and its importance: staying hydrated throughout the day

Chapter 3: Exercise and Physical Activity

- Finding the right exercise routine: cardio, strength training, and flexibility

- Incorporating physical activity into daily life: walking, stairs, and household chores

- Listening to your body: avoiding overtraining and injuries

Chapter 4: Mind-Body Connection

- Stress management techniques: meditation, deep breathing, and yoga

- The role of sleep in weight loss: getting enough quality rest

- Positive mindset and motivation: overcoming challenges and setbacks

Chapter 5: Healthy Eating Habits

- Grocery shopping tips: choosing healthy foods and avoiding processed products

- Mindful eating: paying attention to hunger and fullness cues

- Balancing meals and snacks: creating a satisfying diet

Chapter 6: Portion Control and Healthy Eating Out

- Understanding portion sizes: using visual cues and measuring tools

- Eating out wisely: making healthy choices at restaurants and food stands

- Healthy alternatives: swaps and substitutions for unhealthy foods

Chapter 7: Weight Loss Challenges and Solutions

- Plateaus and how to break through them: adjusting your routine and mindset

- Emotional eating: managing stress and emotional triggers

- Social support and accountability: finding a support system and staying motivated

Chapter 8: Measuring Progress and Celebrating Success

- Tracking your progress: using a food diary, fitness tracker, and measuring tape

- Celebrating milestones: rewarding yourself for achievements

- Staying committed to your goals: maintaining a healthy lifestyle long-term

Chapter 9: Maintaining Weight Loss

- Lifestyle changes for long-term success: incorporating healthy habits into your daily routine

- Avoiding weight regain: being mindful of your eating and exercise habits

- Seeking professional support: consulting a healthcare provider or registered dietitian

Chapter 10: Inspiring Stories and Tips

- Real-life weight loss journeys: success stories and lessons learned

- Additional resources and tips: books, websites, and apps for weight loss

- Embracing a healthier, happier you: celebrating your transformation and enjoying the benefits

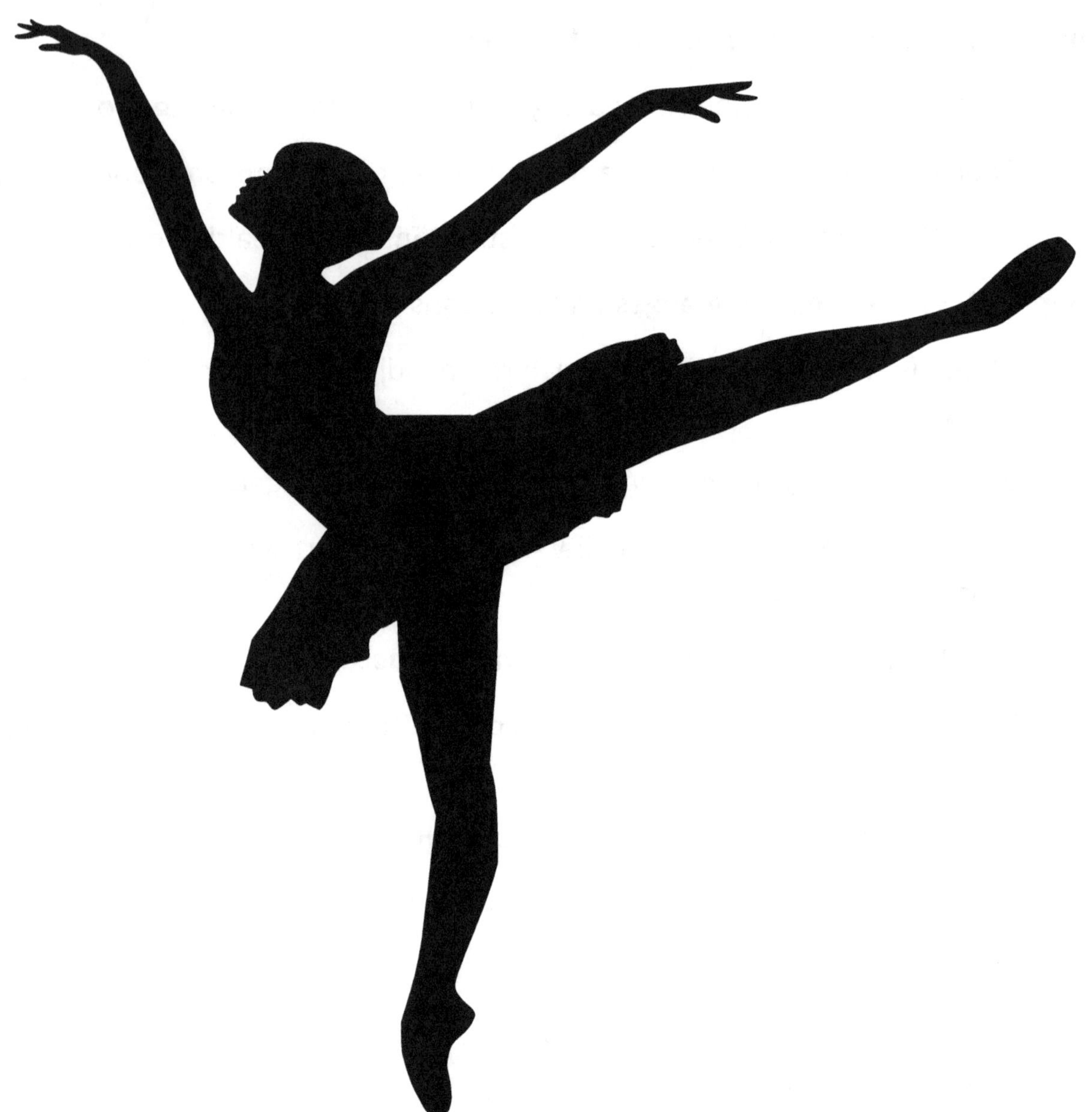

- **"Don't let yesterday use up too much of today."** – Unknown

- **"The body achieves what the mind believes."** - Unknown

- **"The only person you need to be better than is your former self."** - Unknown

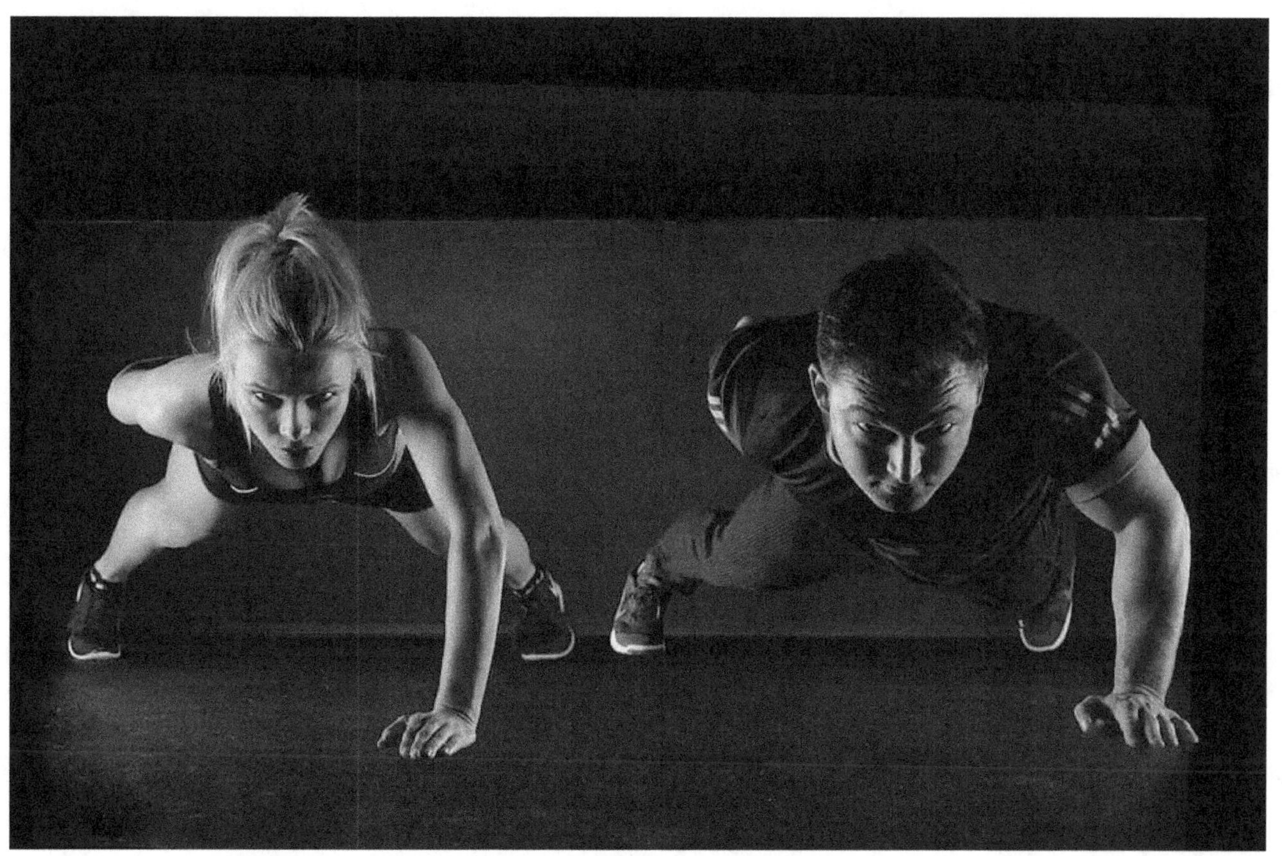

- "Start where you are. Use what you have. Do what you can." - Arthur Ashe

- "Fitness is not a destination, it's a way of life." - Unknown

- "The pain you feel today will be the strength you feel tomorrow." - Unknown

Chapter 1: Understanding Weight Loss

The Science of Weight Loss

Weight loss is a complex process influenced by various factors, including metabolism, calorie intake, and hormonal balance. Understanding the science behind weight loss can help you make informed decisions and develop a sustainable plan.

Metabolism

Metabolism is the rate at which your body burns calories. It's influenced by factors such as age, gender, muscle mass, and activity level. A higher metabolism means you burn more calories, making it easier to lose weight.

Calories

To lose weight, you need to consume fewer calories than you burn. This creates a calorie deficit that forces your body to tap into stored fat for energy. However, it's important to note that drastic calorie restriction can be harmful and unsustainable.

Hormones

Hormones play a significant role in weight management. Hormones like leptin and ghrelin regulate hunger and fullness, while insulin affects how your body stores and uses glucose. Hormonal imbalances can contribute to weight gain or difficulty losing weight.

Setting Realistic Goals

Setting realistic goals is essential for successful weight loss. They should be specific, measurable, achievable, relevant, and time-bound (SMART). Here's how to set effective goals:

- **Short-term goals:** These are smaller, more achievable goals that can help you stay motivated. For example, you might aim to lose 5 pounds in a month.

- **Long-term goals:** These are your ultimate weight loss targets. They should be challenging but attainable. For instance, you might want to lose 20 pounds and maintain a healthy weight.

Overcoming Common Misconceptions

There are many misconceptions about weight loss that can lead to frustration and disappointment. Here are some common myths to avoid:

- **Fad diets:** These diets often promise quick results but are typically unsustainable and unhealthy. They can lead to nutrient deficiencies and weight regain.

- **Quick fixes:** There is no magic pill or quick fix for weight loss. Sustainable weight loss requires consistent effort and lifestyle changes.

- **All calories are created equal:** The quality of your calories matters. Nutrient-dense foods provide essential nutrients and keep you feeling full, while processed foods are often high in calories and low in nutrients.

By understanding the science of weight loss, setting realistic goals, and dispelling common misconceptions, you can create a sustainable and effective weight loss plan. Remember, weight loss is a journey, not a destination. Patience, perseverance, and a healthy approach are key to achieving your goals.

Chapter 2: Making Lifestyle Changes

Nutrition Basics

A healthy diet is essential for weight loss and overall well-being. Understanding the basics of nutrition can help you make informed choices about the foods you eat.

Macronutrients

Macronutrients are the building blocks of your diet. They provide energy and support bodily functions. The three main macronutrients are:

- **Carbohydrates:** They are the primary source of energy for your body. Complex carbohydrates, found in whole grains, fruits, and vegetables, are more nutritious than simple carbohydrates, found in processed foods.

- **Protein:** Protein is essential for building and repairing tissues. It is found in lean meats, poultry, fish, eggs, dairy products, beans, and lentils.

- **Fat:** Healthy fats, found in avocados, nuts, seeds, and olive oil, are essential for nutrient absorption and hormone production. Avoid unhealthy fats, such as saturated and trans fats.

Micronutrients

Micronutrients are vitamins and minerals that your body needs in small amounts. They support various bodily functions, including immune system health, energy production, and cell growth. Good sources of micronutrients include fruits, vegetables, whole grains, lean meats, and dairy products.

Portion Control

Eating the right amount of food is crucial for weight loss. Portion control involves being mindful of how much you eat and avoiding overeating. Using smaller plates, measuring portions, and listening to your body's hunger and fullness cues can help you manage portion sizes.

Meal Planning and Preparation

Meal planning and preparation can help you stay on track with your healthy eating goals. By planning your meals in advance and preparing them ahead of time, you can avoid unhealthy impulse choices and save time.

Healthy Recipes

There are countless healthy recipes available online and in cookbooks. Experiment with different cuisines and ingredients to find dishes that you enjoy. Incorporate a variety of fruits, vegetables, whole grains, lean proteins, and healthy fats into your meals.

Time-Saving Tips

- **Batch cooking:** Prepare large quantities of meals or ingredients on the weekends and store them in the refrigerator or freezer for easy reheating.

- **Meal prepping:** Assemble your meals or snacks in advance so they are ready to grab and go.

- **Using a slow cooker:** Slow cookers are great for preparing healthy, hands-off meals.

- **Having healthy snacks on hand:** Keep a variety of healthy snacks, such as fruits, vegetables, nuts, seeds, or Greek yogurt, readily available.

Hydration and Its Importance

Staying hydrated is essential for overall health and can also support weight loss. Drinking enough water helps regulate your metabolism, aids in digestion, and can reduce feelings of hunger.

How Much Water to Drink

The amount of water you need to drink varies depending on factors such as your activity level, climate, and overall health. A general guideline is to aim for at least 8 glasses of water per day.

Signs of Dehydration

- Thirst

- Dry mouth

- Fatigue

- Dizziness

- Headache

- Dark urine

By making healthy choices and incorporating meal planning and preparation into your lifestyle, you can create a sustainable approach to weight loss. Remember, small changes can make a big difference over time.

Sources and related content:

www.caloriedetail.com

atonce.com

Chapter 3: Exercise and Physical Activity

Finding the Right Exercise Routine

Regular physical activity is essential for weight loss, improving overall health, and boosting energy levels. The key to finding an effective exercise routine is to choose activities that you enjoy and can stick with.

Cardiovascular Exercise

Cardiovascular exercise, also known as cardio, helps improve heart health, burn calories, and increase endurance. Some popular forms of cardio include:

- **Running:** Running is a high-intensity workout that can help you burn a significant number of calories.
- **Swimming:** Swimming is a low-impact exercise that is gentle on the joints.
- **Cycling:** Cycling is a great way to get outdoors and enjoy the scenery while burning calories.
- **Dancing:** Dancing is a fun and enjoyable way to get your heart rate up.

Strength Training

Strength training helps build muscle mass, which can boost your metabolism and help you burn more calories. It also improves bone density and can reduce the risk of injuries. Some effective strength training exercises include:

- **Weightlifting:** Using weights or resistance bands can help build strength and muscle.
- **Bodyweight exercises:** Push-ups, squats, and lunges are effective bodyweight exercises that can be done anywhere.
- **Yoga:** Yoga combines strength training with flexibility and balance.

Flexibility Training

Flexibility training helps improve your range of motion and reduce the risk of injuries. It can also help improve posture and balance. Some effective flexibility exercises include:

- **Stretching:** Static stretching involves holding a stretch for a prolonged period, while dynamic stretching involves moving through a range of motion.

- **Yoga:** Yoga is a great way to improve flexibility and balance.

- **Pilates:** Pilates is a low-impact exercise that focuses on core strength and flexibility.

Incorporating Physical Activity into Daily Life

In addition to structured exercise, there are many ways to incorporate physical activity into your daily life. Here are some ideas:

- **Walking:** Take a walk around the neighborhood or a local park.

- **Taking the stairs:** Instead of taking the elevator, use the stairs whenever possible.

- **Household chores:** Doing household chores can be a surprisingly effective way to burn calories.

- **Active commuting:** Consider walking, biking, or taking public transportation to work or school.

Listening to Your Body

It's important to listen to your body and avoid overtraining. Overtraining can lead to injuries, fatigue, and a decrease in motivation. Pay attention to your body's signals and take rest days when needed.

Signs of Overtraining

- Persistent fatigue

- Decreased performance

- Increased heart rate

- Difficulty sleeping

- Frequent injuries

By finding the right exercise routine, incorporating physical activity into your daily life, and listening to your body, you can achieve your weight loss goals and improve your overall health. Remember, consistency is key to long-term success.

Sources and related content

physiorehabsolution.com

Chapter 4: Mind-Body Connection

Stress Management Techniques

Stress can have a significant impact on weight loss. When you're stressed, you may be more likely to reach for unhealthy comfort foods or engage in emotional eating. Effective stress management techniques can help you cope with stress in a healthy way.

Meditation

Meditation is a powerful tool for reducing stress and promoting relaxation. It involves focusing your attention on your breath or a mantra. Regular meditation can help calm your mind, reduce anxiety, and improve overall well-being.

Deep Breathing

Deep breathing exercises can help activate the body's relaxation response. By taking slow, deep breaths, you can reduce stress and improve your mood.

Yoga

Yoga combines physical postures, breathing exercises, and meditation to promote relaxation and reduce stress. It can also improve flexibility, balance, and strength.

The Role of Sleep in Weight Loss

Getting enough quality sleep is essential for weight loss. When you're sleep-deprived, your body's hormones that regulate hunger and fullness can become unbalanced, leading to increased cravings and overeating.

Tips for Improving Sleep

- Create a relaxing bedtime routine
- Avoid caffeine and alcohol before bed
- Ensure your bedroom is dark, quiet, and cool
- Stick to a consistent sleep schedule

Positive Mindset and Motivation

A positive mindset can play a crucial role in your weight loss journey. It can help you stay motivated, overcome challenges, and believe in your ability to succeed.

Overcoming Challenges and Setbacks

Everyone experiences setbacks on their weight loss journey. It's important to learn from these setbacks and use them as opportunities for growth. Here are some tips for overcoming challenges:

- **Set realistic expectations:** Remember that weight loss is a gradual process. Don't expect to see immediate results.

- **Celebrate small victories:** Acknowledge your progress, no matter how small.

- **Find a support system:** Surround yourself with people who support and encourage you.

- **Stay positive:** Focus on the benefits of your healthy lifestyle, rather than the weight loss itself.

By managing stress, getting enough sleep, and maintaining a positive mindset, you can improve your overall well-being and increase your chances of achieving your weight loss goals. Remember, it's important to be patient and kind to yourself throughout this journey.

Sources and related content

casadesante.com

Chapter 5: Healthy Eating Habits

Grocery Shopping Tips

Choosing healthy foods at the grocery store can be challenging, especially with the abundance of processed and packaged products. Here are some tips for making healthy choices:

- **Read labels carefully:** Pay attention to ingredients, serving sizes, and nutritional information. Look for foods that are low in added sugars, unhealthy fats, and sodium.

- **Focus on the perimeter:** The perimeter of the grocery store typically has fresh produce, meat, poultry, fish, and dairy products.

- **Choose whole grains:** Opt for whole grains over refined grains, which are often processed and stripped of nutrients.

- **Buy in bulk:** Purchasing items in bulk can save you money and reduce food waste.

- **Avoid processed foods:** Processed foods are often high in unhealthy fats, sugars, and sodium. Stick to whole, unprocessed foods whenever possible.

Mindful Eating

Mindful eating involves paying attention to your body's hunger and fullness cues. It can help you avoid overeating and make healthier food choices.

- **Listen to your body:** Pay attention to your hunger and fullness signals. Eat when you're hungry and stop eating when you're satisfied.

- **Eat slowly:** Take your time to savor your food and enjoy the experience.

- **Avoid distractions:** Turn off your phone and TV while eating to focus on your meal.

- **Practice gratitude:** Express gratitude for the food you are eating.

Balancing Meals and Snacks

A balanced diet includes a variety of foods from all food groups. It's important to balance your meals and snacks to ensure you're getting the nutrients your body needs.

- **Eat a balanced breakfast:** Start your day with a nutritious breakfast that includes protein, carbohydrates, and healthy fats.

- **Have regular meals:** Aim to eat every 3-4 hours to avoid feeling overly hungry.

- **Choose healthy snacks:** Opt for snacks that are high in fiber and protein, such as fruits, vegetables, nuts, or Greek yogurt.

- **Control portion sizes:** Pay attention to portion sizes to avoid overeating.

By following these tips, you can develop healthy eating habits that will support your weight loss goals and improve your overall health. Remember, sustainable weight loss is about making long-term lifestyle changes, not following short-term fads.

Understanding Portion Sizes

Portion control is essential for weight management. Understanding portion sizes can help you eat the right amount of food and avoid overeating.

Visual Cues

Using visual cues can help you estimate portion sizes without using measuring tools. Here are some helpful guidelines:

- **Your palm:** Your palm can be used to estimate a portion of protein, such as meat, poultry, or fish.

- **Your fist:** Your fist can be used to estimate a portion of vegetables.

- **Your cupped hand:** Your cupped hand can be used to estimate a portion of grains, such as rice, pasta, or quinoa.

Measuring Tools

If you want to be more precise, you can use measuring tools to portion out your food. Common measuring tools include:

- **Measuring cups and spoons:** These are useful for measuring ingredients for recipes.

- **Food scale:** A food scale can help you measure portions accurately.

- **Portion control plates:** These plates are divided into sections to help you control portion sizes.

Eating Out Wisely

Eating out can be challenging when trying to maintain a healthy diet. However, with a little planning and knowledge, you can make healthy choices at restaurants and food stands.

- **Read menus carefully:** Look for items that are grilled, baked, or steamed, and avoid those that are fried or breaded.

- **Choose wisely:** Opt for salads, soups, grilled fish or chicken, or lean protein dishes.

- **Ask for modifications:** Don't be afraid to ask for modifications to your meal, such as omitting unhealthy toppings or sauces.

- **Control portion sizes:** Be mindful of portion sizes when eating out. Consider sharing a meal or taking some home for later.

Healthy Alternatives

There are many healthy alternatives to unhealthy foods that you can enjoy. Here are some examples:

- **Instead of fried food:** Choose grilled, baked, or roasted options.

- **Instead of sugary drinks:** Opt for water, unsweetened tea, or sparkling water with a squeeze of lemon or lime.

- **Instead of processed snacks:** Choose fruits, vegetables, nuts, or Greek yogurt.

- **Instead of heavy sauces:** Ask for sauces on the side or choose a lighter sauce.

By understanding portion sizes, eating out wisely, and making healthy substitutions, you can maintain a healthy diet even when you're on the go. Remember, it's all about making informed choices and enjoying your food in moderation.

Plateaus and How to Break Through Them

Hitting a plateau in your weight loss journey can be frustrating. However, it's important to remember that plateaus are a common occurrence. Here are some strategies to help you break through a plateau:

- **Re-evaluate your routine:** If you haven't seen results in several weeks, it might be time to reassess your exercise routine or diet. Consider increasing the intensity of your workouts or making adjustments to your meal plan.

- **Track your progress:** Keep a food diary and exercise log to track your intake and activity levels. This can help you identify any areas where you need to make changes.

- **Increase your activity:** Try adding more physical activity to your routine, such as taking a brisk walk or doing some light cardio.

- **Be patient:** Breaking through a plateau takes time. Don't get discouraged if you don't see immediate results.

Emotional Eating

Emotional eating is when you use food to cope with stress, boredom, or other negative emotions. It can be a challenge to overcome, but with the right strategies, you can manage emotional eating and stay on track with your weight loss goals.

- **Identify your triggers:** Pay attention to the situations or emotions that lead you to emotional eating.

- **Find healthy coping mechanisms:** Develop healthy ways to manage stress, such as meditation, exercise, or spending time with loved ones.

- **Practice mindful eating:** Pay attention to your hunger and fullness cues, and avoid eating when you're not truly hungry.

- **Seek support:** Talk to a friend, family member, or therapist about your emotional eating challenges.

Social Support and Accountability

Having a strong support system can make a big difference in your weight loss journey. Surrounding yourself with people who support and encourage you can help you stay motivated and accountable.

- **Find a support group:** Join a weight loss support group or online community.

- **Involve a friend or family member:** Ask a friend or family member to join you on your weight loss journey.

- **Hire a personal trainer or nutritionist:** A professional can provide guidance, support, and accountability.

- **Celebrate your successes:** Reward yourself for achieving your goals, no matter how small.

Remember, weight loss is a journey, not a destination. It's important to be patient, persistent, and kind to yourself. By addressing challenges and seeking support, you can overcome obstacles and achieve your weight loss goals.

Chapter 8: Measuring Progress and Celebrating Success

Tracking Your Progress

Tracking your progress is an important part of any weight loss journey. It can help you stay motivated, identify areas where you need to make changes, and celebrate your successes.

- **Keep a food diary:** Record everything you eat and drink, including portion sizes. This can help you identify any unhealthy eating habits.

- **Track your exercise:** Keep a record of your workouts, including the type of activity, duration, and intensity.

- **Measure your body:** Measure your weight, waist circumference, and other relevant measurements regularly.

- **Take progress photos:** Take photos of yourself at regular intervals to see your physical transformation.

Celebrating Milestones

Celebrating your successes is essential for staying motivated and maintaining your progress. Even small victories can be a big deal.

- **Set small, achievable goals:** Break down your larger goals into smaller, more manageable steps.

- **Reward yourself:** Treat yourself to something you enjoy when you reach a milestone.

- **Share your progress:** Share your successes with friends, family, or your support group.

Staying Committed to Your Goals

Staying committed to your weight loss goals can be challenging, especially when you encounter setbacks. Here are some tips for staying motivated:

- **Focus on the benefits:** Remind yourself of the reasons why you want to lose weight. Think about how it will improve your health, energy levels, and overall quality of life.

- **Find a workout buddy:** Having a workout buddy can make it more fun and enjoyable to exercise.

- **Don't give up:** Even if you slip up, don't give up on your goals. Everyone makes mistakes. Just pick yourself up and keep going.

- **Seek professional help:** If you're struggling to stay motivated or make progress, consider talking to a therapist, nutritionist, or personal trainer.

By tracking your progress, celebrating your successes, and staying committed to your goals, you can achieve your weight loss dreams. Remember, it's a journey, not a destination. Enjoy the process and celebrate your accomplishments along the way.

Chapter 9: Maintaining Weight Loss

Lifestyle Changes for Long-Term Success

Once you've achieved your weight loss goals, it's important to make sustainable lifestyle changes to maintain your weight. This involves incorporating healthy habits into your daily routine.

- **Healthy eating:** Continue to follow a balanced diet that includes plenty of fruits, vegetables, whole grains, lean protein, and healthy fats.

- **Regular exercise:** Aim for at least 150 minutes of moderate-intensity exercise per week.

- **Mindful eating:** Pay attention to your hunger and fullness cues to avoid overeating.

- **Stress management:** Practice stress management techniques, such as meditation, deep breathing, or yoga.

- **Sufficient sleep:** Aim for 7-9 hours of quality sleep each night.

Avoiding Weight Regain

Once you've lost weight, it's important to be mindful of your eating and exercise habits to avoid weight regain. Here are some tips:

- **Monitor your weight:** Weigh yourself regularly to track your progress and catch any signs of weight gain early.

- **Be mindful of portion sizes:** Continue to pay attention to portion sizes and avoid overeating.

- **Stay active:** Maintain a regular exercise routine to burn calories and build muscle.

- **Avoid unhealthy habits:** Limit your consumption of processed foods, sugary drinks, and alcohol.

- **Seek support:** Surround yourself with people who support your healthy lifestyle.

Seeking Professional Support

If you're struggling to maintain your weight loss or have any concerns about your health, it's important to seek professional support. A healthcare provider or registered dietitian can offer guidance and advice.

- **Consult a healthcare provider:** Regular check-ups with your doctor can help monitor your health and identify any potential issues.

- **See a registered dietitian:** A registered dietitian can provide personalized nutrition advice and help you develop a healthy eating plan.

- **Consider a therapist:** If you're struggling with emotional eating or other psychological factors, a therapist can help you address these issues.

By making sustainable lifestyle changes, being mindful of your eating and exercise habits, and seeking professional support when needed, you can maintain your weight loss and enjoy a healthier, happier life. Remember, it's a journey, not a destination.

Sources and related content

curecorner.in

Chapter 10: Inspiring Stories and Tips

Real-Life Weight Loss Journeys

Hearing the stories of others who have successfully lost weight can be inspiring and motivating. In this chapter, we will share real-life weight loss journeys and the lessons learned along the way.

- **Overcoming challenges:** Discover how individuals overcame obstacles, such as plateaus, emotional eating, and lack of motivation.

- **Finding support:** Learn how people found support systems that helped them stay on track.

- **Celebrating success:** Explore how individuals celebrated their achievements and maintained their weight loss.

Additional Resources and Tips

There are many resources available to help you on your weight loss journey. This chapter will provide recommendations for books, websites, and apps that can offer guidance, support, and inspiration.

- **Books:** Discover popular weight loss books that offer practical advice and motivation.

- **Websites:** Explore informative websites that provide tips, recipes, and workout ideas.

- **Apps:** Learn about helpful apps that can track your progress, provide meal plans, and offer exercise routines.

Embracing a Healthier, Happier You

Once you've achieved your weight loss goals, it's time to celebrate your transformation and enjoy the benefits of a healthier lifestyle.

- **Celebrate your achievements:** Acknowledge your hard work and dedication.

- **Focus on the benefits:** Enjoy the improved energy levels, increased confidence, and better overall health that comes with weight loss.

- **Continue to make healthy choices:** Maintain a balanced diet and regular exercise to sustain your weight loss.

- **Inspire others:** Share your journey with others to encourage them on their own weight loss paths.

By reading inspiring stories, utilizing additional resources, and embracing your transformation, you can continue to thrive on your weight loss journey. Remember, it's a lifelong commitment to a healthier, happier you.

Conclusion

This book has provided you with the knowledge and tools you need to embark on a successful weight loss journey. By understanding the science of weight loss, making sustainable lifestyle changes, and seeking support, you can achieve your goals and improve your overall health.

Remember, weight loss is a journey, not a destination. It's important to be patient, persistent, and kind to yourself along the way. Celebrate your successes, learn from your setbacks, and enjoy the process of transforming your life.

With dedication and commitment, you can achieve a healthier, happier you.